BE Free

Stop Smoking

21st Century - Hypnosis

Self Speak Solutions

Carol Cumpston, BS, CCHT

Printed in the United States of America
ISBN 9798740818238

WHY YOU SHOULD READ THIS BOOK

Over 24 million people have a disease related to smoking. You can maximize your potential and become the successful you by using the proven non-evasive method of self-hypnosis to stop smoking.

How a self-healing script can help you to eliminate the smoking habit from the comfort of your own home. As well as, eliminate common problems that can keep you suffering while increasing your self-confidence. Option to record your own powerful voice using the scripts provided. A safe and easy way to get rid of your habit. There are three sessions. Two for smoking and a bonus script for weight control.

A special thanks to Drs. Art & Pam Winkler for the superior training, resources and heartfelt guidance all these years that played a role in my life toward fulfilling my purpose.

I appreciate all my clients who have taught me much about how powerful they are in resolving challenges by allowing me to work with them and the belief they have in themselves.

And special gratitude to my daughter for her years of encouragement and loving support.

CONTENTS

PREFACE

The foundation of Self Speak Solutions is about claiming your personal power and taking responsibility to overcome challenges.

Self Speak Solutions is written under the premise that there is a solution to every problem. These solutions are needed for the physical, mental, emotional and spiritual burdens being felt in a hectic world. We offer resources that inspire and empower you to live your best life.

As an opening to Self Speak Solutions it would be useful to briefly understand the power of suggestion and the workings of the mind. Two levels of mind, the conscious and subconscious mind, are being spoken too. Most of us are cognitively aware of the conscious mind which operates through our senses and develops our perception. This awareness includes what we see, hear, feel and even speak to ourselves. We are all influenced rightly or wrongly by the written words we see, the emotions we feel and sounds we hear.

The subconscious mind records both positive and negative suggestions. The fact is the more emotional our experience is, the more imbedded the suggestion becomes within our psyche and usually without your conscious knowledge causing both pleasant and unpleasant experiences in your life.

So, if someone tells you that you are a wimp while in fact you are very strong, the subconscious mind acts upon the word "wimp" and this weakens your resolve. Making changes through the subconscious mind corrects this. These self speak sessions help you get back your power as you can realize the healing necessary to put your own strengths into action.

How to tap into your inherent subconscious mind can be done easily with the proper guidance. Using carefully worded suggestions, while you focus your attention, can be done in the form of self-healing techniques, imagery, and visualization and more until the desired changes become stronger than the negative information stored in the subconscious mind replacing them with uplifting, loving ideas, emotions and thoughts always during this session.

Your conscious awareness of the progress of these changes may be very subtle to your conscious mind. Eventually, you begin to realize that something seems different and very good. Now you have the opportunity to relax into self-healing just by participating in your life.

INTRODUCTION

Congratulations on your decision to become a happy, healthy, energetic non-smoker. This script is easy to use, has updated information and represents two complete individual sessions. Now you can experience the benefits personally in your own home just by following the directions I am giving you. You begin to realize and believe that being a clean air breather is a great opportunity to live your life to its fullest… as your resolve is more powerful than ever.

Whenever you listen to each meditative session you enjoy the good feelings of being a non-smoker and everlasting peacefulness. Listening seven days in a row can help make the changes more permanent and attainable. Repeating each session makes the suggestions even stronger each time by increasing your intention. Thereafter, listen whenever you feel you could use reinforcement. Clients have proven that there are different times a person quits smoking. I have had clients quit immediately, at several weeks or more. Your response time is personal to you. Practicing good habits replaces the old harmful ones such as not purchasing smoking products. You, also, experience higher vibrating power and choose more beneficial habits like exercising and eating right.

 It is recommended you record this session on your phone or computer. Allow 25 minutes for your recording. Record only the words within the quotes. Your own voice adds a powerful dimension to your experience. Speak normally and gently at a regular natural pace within the quotes. When you see these dots … you simply take a new breath then continue. You can also choose someone reliable to help you by reading the script to you in a quiet peaceful setting. Use of a chair or bed to support your relaxed body in a bedroom or office is preferred.

The importance of reading these suggestions as specifically written is of great importance. Changing or rearranging any words can change the meaning to the subconscious mind weakening its intention. Please do follow these instructions completely. NEVER listen to this session while in a car but enjoy a peaceful calm environment instead.

People have been searching for a natural way to quit smoking. Everyone desires to get rid of bad habits. You now have an opportunity to get rid of the smoking habit using your own inherent abilities and wisdom to quit smoking with the proper guidance.

 Do you want a lasting state of peace and well-being? Are you willing to experience a more profound and easy way to quit smoking?   If you can answer yes you are ready to begin this self-healing session! You will notice how much you expand your awareness and feel peace from within during your self-healing session and thereafter.

 There is nothing your conscious mind needs to do as the subconscious mind records all the information you say and makes it true. Allow your inner spirit to assist in your intention to quit smoking now.

"Allow yourself to get comfortable in your favorite relaxed position... and raise your eyes up to the ceiling holding for 10 seconds... as you now close your eyes... while breathing deeply into your heart... and with each out breath you take, you spontaneously go deeper relaxed... as you release each breath all tension dissipates from your being... stretch your entire body before you go into a deep state of relaxation...and then again take a deep cleansing breath and with each out breath just let go of all stress and strain as you feel like a burden, a heavy weight has been expelled from your being... as the muscles in and around your eyes relax all by themselves... and becoming more peaceful and secure... as your relaxation becomes multiplied and magnified... and you continue relaxing down deeper your chin lowers toward your chest... and your breath sends a message of acceptance and renewal to your consciousness and cells similar to dominoes in action... and each cell transfers a message to the next about your deep relaxation... becoming much more calm and tranquil...as you expand your inner awareness."

"And all sounds and noises simply cause you to become drowsier... and my voice takes you into the perfect level of healing relaxation for you...as you now feel safer and secure... (Pause 5 seconds) and continue to relax more and more as you scan your body for any area that may remain tense... (Pause 5 seconds) if you find any tension, then focus on that area and tighten it, then silently count to 5 then let go, as you automatically let the tension go away (Pause 5 seconds)… as the subconscious mind hears each word I say… and you will be pleasantly surprised with your continuous progress as a clean air breather."

"As you continue to be relaxed, comfortable and secure… feeling more empowered as you let your inner mind float freely…and envision or image that you are slowly walking around a shopping mall… and observe the colors and shapes… as you look down below you notice 2 levels… and you see a store you would like to explore down on the lowest level… you move to an glass encased escalator traveling down slowly and easily… as you notice all the sights below… as you continue to move further down to the bottom level… and you listen to the pleasant sounds around you… and on your left you notice a small tree with 8 gifts underneath and you begin counting backwards down to the number 1 like this… 8… 7… 6…5…4…3…2…1 counting to yourself as you go deeper down to the lowest level…and you reach this level you feel very calm, at peace and serene… while going deeper and deeper down… as you now have reached the perfect level of healing relaxation for your instant changes… because you feel so good as you have made it down safely."

"Just enjoy the feeling of relaxation in your body and mind now… as you allow this relaxation it brings about a strong feeling of peaceful confidence within you… because you have released all inner tension… because that tension in your body weakens your energy and whatever has held you back from the past… and now this is your moment, your place to be calm with clarity of mind… because there is nothing your conscious mind need to do… while your body and mind are now relaxed and open to accept all the benefits from the suggestions I give you… connecting with your oneness… and staying in touch with your inner feelings frees you like an eagle flying across the universe… and you realize it is okay to accept whatever feelings you have because you have to acknowledge them first in order to change any negative feelings… you can feel good about this understanding… fully accepting all new information that helps you to create new habits that increase your level of being healthy and content."

Water Signal

"I'm going to tell you a signal now that will begin working today and will continue working for the rest of your life… the unconscious levels of your mind will cause the signal to work."

"The signal is water, and here is how the unconscious levels of your mind will cause it to work."

"From now on, for the rest of your life, every time you look at water, the unconscious levels of your mind and all levels of your inner mind will cooperate and cause you to become relaxed, and calm, and peaceful… every time you look at water your nerves become more relaxed and steady, and you continue becoming more calm emotionally… any water you look at is an automatic signal, including rain, puddles of water, water coming out of a faucet, water in a shower or a bathtub, water in a swimming pool, a pond, a creek, a river, a lake or in the ocean…"

"Being more calm and relaxed and that enables you to think more clearly… it enables you to focus your attention more readily… and you will be able to concentrate better… that causes your memory to keep improving… you will also find that being more calm and relaxed causes all of your body processes and activities to continue functioning more perfectly… and that cause your health to keep improving more each day… you will be pleased to find yourself experiencing many other really wonderful benefits…"

"Your pancreas, your kidneys, your liver, your heart, and all other organs and glands in your body will continue functioning more perfectly."

"Your immune system, your digestive system, your assimilation system, your blood pressure system, your metabolism, your elimination system, all continue functioning more perfectly, and your health continues improving more each day."

"From now on for the rest of your life, every time you look at water, your mind will cause you to become relaxed, calm and feel peaceful, and you will remain calm, relaxed and peaceful for at least eight hours every time you look at water… That will keep you calm and relaxed as you go about your daily activities… You will have more energy, more strength and vitality, and you will continue becoming more efficient in your work and other activities from being more relaxed and more at ease."

1 (Dr. E. Arthur Winkler, page 14, Hypnotic Inductions and Prescriptions)

"Allow my voice to guide you now, as you silently say these words to yourself.   From this day forward I have discontinued any urge or craving to smoke... and I have already discontinued any and all interest in smoking... because I have taken this action to change... because I realize avoidance is the true reason I smoked... as smoking is only a shift of responsibility that takes away my power... but smoking really causes harm to me... now as I have quit smoking, I become in control of my life again... and I become more efficient in my work... I feel and look more attractive... I am more optimistic, confident, independent, healthy and energetic... and I maintain an inner sense of security... because I now understand that it is an untrue belief that cigarette smoking has any power over me... because I now discontinue my false belief of security in smoking... as being a clean air breather who now acts responsibly ... because I deserve better... and I have inner courage and I always use my own power to help me as it is a matter of my life or death... and I have made a commitment to respect and protect my body... because I love myself and my family... and I am a clean air breather... and I live in a state of peace and well-being."

"Continue to remain calm and relaxed... as this session helps eliminate the desire and cravings for smoking products... because you have decided to quit smoking without any uncomfortable side effects... as that allows you the freedom from withdrawal symptoms... and cigarettes automatically disappear from your mind the moment you see them or think of them... because they have discontinued being part of your life... and because of this you have become happier and healthier..."

"And you stop using food as a substitute… and you eat only when you are truly hungry and when your body needs nourishment… as you have developed the good habit of eating smaller portions and less fat and sugar… and you always ignore any suggestions to put a cigarette in your hand or mouth, whether you are drinking, eating or socializing… because you cooperate with your subconscious mind and prefer healthier outlets for your stress… such as deep breathing…. And that easily calms your mind… as you relax without worry…and you always remember just taking a few minutes to be with your authentic loving self…"

"As you calmly continue to relax deeper down… because being born with conscious responsibility lets you have complete control over your life and how you act… as having a choice is one of the most powerful attributes you have… and you have now chosen to improve your life by responding to daily stress calmly without smoking… as you take careful thought out actions, instead of reacting emotionally… and whenever your body tightens because of stress it weakens your immune system, endangering your health… leaving your immune system unable to fight off viruses, bacteria and other illnesses and diseases… as you have instead chosen to intentional act with calmness and clear thoughts… and you always remember you are a clean air breather… because this is where true happiness resides within you."

"And you believe that now you are a non-smoker… you have made a commitment to respect and protect your body and mind… as you think and act as a non-smoker… because you make this commitment spontaneously on a daily basis… and you feel good about yourself… because having an inner sense of gratitude increases your healing power… and you realize now that all your goals are so much closer and easier than ever before… and this is so." Let me tell you a story.

"Have you ever wondered how it is that when you drive you automatically… and without conscious effort change your direction, especially to avoid an accident?… and truthfully when you first learn to drive, initially you use your conscious mind to perform your actions… and at that moment you consciously think about controlling and directing the car… as when to put on the brakes to stop and when to accelerate to go forward… and if you continue to practice all these movements eventually, without conscious effort, the movements become automatic… because these movements have become programmed into your subconscious mind… and likewise as you continue to venture out onto the road with your car, you follow along automatically… and if changes were made to improve the road… then again you easily adjust your mind and effortlessly relearn your new direction, calmly and without hesitation… because it is wiser for you to do this… and this improved pattern become spontaneous and easy… as these corrections reside both within your conscious and subconscious mind."

"The information in the storehouse of your mind that has been causing that problem is based on misunderstandings in the subconscious part of your mind… The subconscious mind can be accessing, reviewing and looking at your problem from a different point of view than it had when it first went into your mind… and is incorporating changes within now knowingly and unknowingly… your subconscious mind is changing those patterns of behavior that have been causing that problem... and is enabling you to develop new patterns of behavior that enable you to be completely free from that problem... and you can be delightfully surprised how easy it is to overcome that problem within a short while… as you continue to adjust your life to whatever brings your highest good."

"Every day in every way you demonstrate integrity in all your actions, being calmer on all levels… as you noticed now how stable and settled you have become… as you will continue to act responsible with great confidence and motivation… and your feelings of happiness are increasing, and your day to day living becomes more pleasurable… as you are rapidly becoming the person you have always secretly been… as your authentic self… because you have become totally self-confident, self-sufficient, healthy, acceptable, capable, balanced and strong,"

"This session is ending in a few moments. After a count from 1 to 5 you will come up to a full alert peaceful state of mind.

1. Every day in every way you are free from the smoking habit. Every time you read or listen to this session you welcome the new habits and skills you have developed.

2. You have renewed your commitment as a clean air breather. Each breath you take increases the good confident feelings within.

3. You feel more in balance, in perfect harmony with your renewed body & emotions and at peace mind, body, heart and soul. Now you are experiencing an everlasting state of gratitude for your wonderfully empowered life.

4. Feeling vibrant, energized and refreshed as you move up to full alertness free from the smoking habit.

5. You can open your eyes with a new sense of joy, profound happiness and contentment."

CHAPTER 2 - STOP SMOKING II

"Before you drift into a dream like peaceful state, have your clothes loosened in any areas where they might feel tight… as now you put yourself into a comfortable position… and noticing the feeling of warmth as your body is supported… and raise your eyes up to the ceiling and hold for 10 seconds... and this allows you to go even more comfortable as you now close your eyes… and take a deep breath… as you can feel the fresh air going into your nose and then down deep into your belly… as you easily hold that breath for 3 seconds and feel yourself relax even more as you gently exhale… and with each out breath you take, you go deeper relaxed as you listen to every word I say… as my voice takes you deeper into the perfect level of healing relaxation for you… and observe your breath now… as you move into your natural state of peacefulness… and you continue to relax and all tension disappears…

And again take a deep cleansing breath... and with each out breath you notice how easy you release all regrets, all resentments, harmful habits and now feeling so much lighter… as you bring your attention to your heart… as you take a moment to feel gratitude for all that it has done for you… and give yourself love and receive love from others… as you take in all these words, all other sounds in your environment fade away now… as you continue relaxing deeper still… and becoming much more connected, comfortable and peaceful… as an unconditional love develops within you effortlessly."

"And you understand what it's like to day dream about something… and not really be listening to anything, while someone in the same room may be talking to you… but instead of hearing them you are visualizing the ocean… or you can be walking slowly on a path into a beautiful forest listening to nature call… or you can be enjoying yourself dancing freely… and you continue day dreaming… (Pause 5 sec.) as your awareness narrows down, to the enjoyable sensations you are experiencing now… and you enjoy dreaming… and in your dreams you can do many wonderful and pleasant things… as you can float on a raft… and you can sway back and forth in a swing… or laugh at a funny movie… or reminisce about a wonderful childhood experience or play at the park… and it is very real that you don't realize you are dreaming…"

"The subconscious part of your mind is an incredible storehouse of memories, ideas and images that help you go into a deep calm inner state… and discover numerous things you can do… and you're capable of doing much more than you have ever been aware of… and you can continue easily to breathe deeply… and do two more deep breathes… as it doesn't really make any difference what your conscious mind does because your subconscious mind can do just what it must do to work out a pleasant solution to your problem."

Water Signal

"I'm going to tell you a signal now that will begin working today and will continue working for the rest of your life… the unconscious levels of your mind will cause the signal to work."

"The signal is water, and here is how the unconscious levels of your mind will cause it to work."

"From now on, for the rest of your life, every time you look at water, the unconscious levels of your mind and all levels of your inner mind will cooperate and cause you to become relaxed, and calm, and peaceful… every time you look at water your nerves become more relaxed and steady, and you continue becoming more calm emotionally… any water you look at is an automatic signal, including rain, puddles of water, water coming out of a faucet, water in a shower or a bathtub, water in a swimming pool, a pond, a creek, a river, a lake or in the ocean…"

"Being more calm and relaxed and that enables you to think more clearly… it enables you to focus your attention more readily… and you will be able to concentrate better… that causes your memory to keep improving… you will also find that being more calm and relaxed causes all of your body processes and activities to continue functioning more perfectly… and that cause your health to keep improving more each day… you will be pleased to find yourself experiencing many other really wonderful benefits…"

"Your pancreas, your kidneys, your liver, your heart, and all other organs and glands in your body will continue functioning more perfectly."

"Your immune system, your digestive system, your assimilation system, your blood pressure system, your metabolism, your elimination system, all continue functioning more perfectly, and your health continues improving more each day."

"From now on for the rest of your life, every time you look at water, your mind will cause you to become relaxed, calm and feel peaceful, and you will remain calm, relaxed and peaceful for at least eight hours every time you look at water… That will keep you calm and relaxed as you go about your daily activities… You will have more energy, more strength and vitality, and you will continue becoming more efficient in your work and other activities from being more relaxed and more at ease."

1 (Dr. E. Arthur Winkler, page 14, Hypnotic Inductions and Prescriptions)

"Now continue to relax deeper down… feeling good, feeling calmer… as you have decided to get rid of the smoking habit… and from this day forward your cravings or desire to smoke tobacco products has been eliminated… because you have easily forgotten what smoking is like… as all smoking and tobacco products have discontinued having any power over you… and in this very moment you are a non-smoker, a clean air breather, healthier and happier every day in every way…"

"Because now you realize that smoking can cause great harm to your body… and people who smoke become susceptible to all kinds of illnesses and disease… from a cold to cancer, heart disease and emphysema… and socially it affects you with discolored teeth and bad breath… smoking causes tooth decay… and shortness of breath…and your clothes smell bad… and you risk getting burn holes in your clothing and personal belongings…"

"And now each day you have more energy and feel free as you are glad you are a non-smoker… and your lungs are healthier, your teeth whiter… as your breath is fresher… and your body and clothes have discontinued smelling like smoke… Your subconscious mind and all inner levels of mind accept these suggestions as being true…"

"Beginning at this very moment you can have a profound sense of well-being, pride and self confidence that you are indeed a non-smoker… and when you awaken in the morning you notice how much more energized you feel… and when others smoke around you, you continue to be a clean air breather…because you dislike the smell of smoke and now feel confident being a clean air breather… and you have complete control over your life, your health… and you can envision your weight at its perfection and ideal weight for you… because that perfect and ideal weight happens since you are a non-smoker… because now the appetite of the mind ceases and stops its present function of overeating… as you eat only what is vital to your body… and eat only when you are truly hungry."

"Because wherever you are, any place, when you observe someone else smoking your realize what is happening to that person… and when you see that person smoking you will feel glad that you are a non-smoker, clean air breather… and you have complete control over your life… and have discontinued being subservient to any poisons or drugs… because now you feel the pride and joy of knowing that you are a non-smoker, clean air breather."

"The subconscious mind can now access, review and look at your problem from a different point of view than it had when it first went into your mind… and is incorporating changes within now knowingly and unknowingly… and you can be delightfully surprised how easy it is to overcome that problem within a short while… as you continue to adjust your new life whatever brings your highest good." "You glow with a wonderful sense of accomplishment… as your inner mind understands what must be done and is working out a solution to that problem now… and you always realize what to do and when to do it… and your self-reliance, self-worth and self-determination become stronger and rewarding every day in every way… and you embrace your life with enthusiasm and love for yourself and others… as patience and persistence now become your new motto, as your spirit is renewed."

(optional) "The subconscious level of your mind is hearing and receiving my suggestions and instructions... and are inspiring you with creative ideas that will strengthen your spirit of enthusiasm for living your life more fully... and your mind is receptive to the joy, and love and peace of God... and you are experiencing greater strength and vitality in your mind, soul and body."

"You have really great capability... Jesus said, 'The kingdom of God is within you...'" This means you have all the strength, power and wisdom you need to achieve your goals in life... and you will continue progressing as you follow a path that leads to happiness and fulfillment...

"Most of the sacred writings reveal that God can and will help you work out ways to have your needs fulfilled... God is an unlimited source of supply... and your awareness of that truth keeps becoming more real to you each day... and it enables you to be open to an inflow and outflow of God's love, peace, joy, happiness and all the other good things that life has to offer."

"God is also the source of perfect health... he created you with amazing healing powers that can keep your body healthy and strong at all times... you realize that God is life, and God's will for you and for everyone is good health, happiness and prosperity... and your faith in those truths keeps becoming strong each day."

"Your mind is at peace... and your faith is continually increasing... each day you keep becoming more optimistic and you see life as a wonderful experience with great opportunities."

"You regard difficulties as an opportunity to experience the power of God working through you... and you see the spirit of God in other people... and realize that they too are on this earth to experience the opportunity to learn and to grow... The right path to take and right decisions to make keep becoming more clear and understandable... and your spirit of love and understanding continue to grow."

"You are a wonderful person and your mind at peace."

2 (Dr. E. Arthur Winkler, page 110, Hypnotic Inductions and Prescription)

"This session is ending in a few moments. After I count from 1 to 5 you will come up to a full alert peaceful state of mind.

1. Every day in every way you are free from the smoking habit. Every time you read or listen to this session you welcome the new habits and skills you have developed.

2. You have renewed your commitment as a clean air breather. Each breath you take increases the good confident feelings within.

3. You feel more in balance, in perfect harmony with your renewed body & emotions and at peace of mind, body, heart and soul. Now you are experiencing an everlasting state of gratitude for your empowered life.

4. Feeling vibrant, energized and refreshed as you move up to full alertness free from the smoking habit.

5. You can open your eyes with a new sense of joy, profound happiness and contentment."

"Allow yourself to get comfortable in your favorite relaxed position… and raise your eyes up to the ceiling holding for 10 seconds… and you now close your eyes… while breathing deeply into your heart… and with each outbreath you take, you spontaneously go deeper relaxed… as you release each breath all tension dissipates from your being… stretch your entire body before you go into a deep state of relaxation… and then again take a deep cleansing breath and with each out breath just let go of all stress and strain as you feel like a burden, a heavy weight has been expelled from your being… as the muscles in and around your eyes relax all by themselves… and becoming more peaceful and secure… as your relaxation becomes multiplied and magnified… and you continue relaxing down deeper as your chin lowers to your chest… and your breath sends a message of acceptance and renewal to your consciousness and cells similar to dominoes in action… and each cell transfers a message to the next about your deep relaxation… becoming much more calm and tranquil… as you expand your inner awareness.

"And all sounds and noises simply cause you to become drowsier… and my voice takes you into the perfect level of healing relaxation for you… as you now feel safer and secure (Pause 5 seconds) and continue to relax more as you scan your body for any area that may remain tense (Pause 5 seconds) if you find any tension, then focus on that area and tighten it, then silently count to 5 then let go as you automatically let the tension go away (Pause 5 seconds)… as the subconscious mind hears each word I say…"

"Just enjoy the feeling of relaxation in your body and mind now… as you allow this relaxation it brings about a strong feeling of peaceful confidence within you… because you have released all inner tension… and now this is your moment, your place to be calm with clarity of mind… because there is nothing your conscious mind need to do… while your body and mind are now relaxed and open to accept all the benefits from the suggestions I give you… connecting with your oneness… and staying in touch with your inner feelings frees you like an eagle flying across the universe… and you realize it is okay to accept whatever feelings you have… because you have to acknowledge them first in order to change any negative feelings… you can feel good about this understanding… fully accepting all new information that helps you to create new habit that increase your level of being healthy and content."

"You have discontinued the urge or emotional need for junk food, and sugary fatty sweets for these are harmful foods without nutritional value, that are depleting your cells of their natural energy… if you decide to snack, then you choose fresh fruits and eating many vegetable all tasting so delicious… and these fruits and vegetables provide you with energy that keep you alert and strong… and you will be eating less and enjoying life more… as you automatically reduce the number of calories you ingest by eating smaller portions… and low saturated fatty foods, eliminating fast foods…"

"Your consistent habit of eating differently causes all unwanted fatty cells and tissues to liquefy so they can easily and safely be eliminated through the proper avenues of your body… and this is a permanent and lasting change… while taking place even when you sleep… and you will be happy to discover yourself reducing from one to two pounds of excess fat a week… as easily, naturally and normally while being permanent and lasting… and physical activity causes you to remove excess body fat safely and effectively forever… as enjoying and accepting your beautiful body and improved self- image… and because you drink plenty of water, you are pleasantly satisfied as your skin becomes softer, more resilient and smoother or your skin becomes silkier, clearer and has more elasticity and radiance or all of these."

"Because each day all of the excess fat continues being eliminated from your body through the natural processes of your elimination system… as you drink fresh, pure water, at least 8 glasses a day… as water balances your cells and keeps your body temperature normal… and most importantly water energizes your brain… and washes away toxins… delicious water becomes your beverage of choice… being very good tasting and satisfying you… and you have now chosen a new lifestyle with perfect balance and correct body fat to muscle ratio for your own body frame and age… as a result your life is reflecting a new reality of harmony, poise and happiness."

"As you create healthy habits, always doing physical activity and exercise on a daily basis just like brushing your teeth… and imagine walking on air while stimulating your cells and metabolism as you use up stored excess fat… and prioritizing those activities into your daily schedule your highest good… and each time you exercise you do so with enthusiasm, flowing in each movement with ease, like having a spring in your step… as you allow good changes to happen to your body automatically… and you are doing that which gives you invigorating and revitalizing energy… as you take in those wonderful and pleasurable changes now… as you relax comfortably, your conscious and subconscious mind are now agreeing that exercise and all safe physical activities are fun, exciting and favorable in your daily life…"

"While you are very comfortable and relaxed I am going to tell you a story that your subconscious mind understands… and this will give you more power to accomplish your weight reduction goals…"

"At some moment in life most people have dreamed of a beautiful new car… as you allow yourself to imagine a beautiful car picture yourself sitting in the driver's seat… as you drive off it's as though your car has always been with you… and being proud of its shiny body, you ride along happily enjoying all the benefits of your journey… this car has a special emergency gas tank that is used only when necessary… and whenever you stop to refuel your car you add just a little more fuel than is needed… and until finally one day you realize your car doesn't drive as efficiently as it used to… and instead it performs as though it were very heavy, slowing down… and you feel stagnant, wondering what to do… then, someone makes you aware of your gas tank that has been filled with excess fuel… and without consciously realizing it you were carrying around a lot of extra and unnecessary fuel… as you realize the ultimate responsibility for taking care of your car belongs to you… and realizing if you leave this excess fuel in the car, your cars performance will continue slowing down… and malfunctioning and eventually prematurely stopping… you must quickly and

effectively get rid of this excess fuel to save your car…
as you wonder how you can get rid of excess fuel…
you decide how effortless it is to use your personal car
for your errands instead of using a delivery service…
and you do this effectively learning how to enjoy the
journey and the movement… and you have your
repairman increase your cars idling speed that it also
reduces more excess fuel much quicker… and even
idling in your driveway the excess fuel goes away and
disappears… and after doing all of this consistently you
notice that your car is in better shape…better than
before… and your car looks and feels good… as if it
was vibrating to a higher energy, smoother, causing
you to think about your own body… then you compare
your body's excess fat to a car with excess fuel in the
tank… finally you understand now that physical activity
uses up stored fat just like your car uses up excess
fuel… and you take advantage of that knowledge and
perform outstandingly."

"This session is ending in a few moments. After a count from 1 to 5 you will come up to a full alert peaceful state of mind.

1. Every time you read or listen to this session you welcome the new habits and skills you have developed.
2. You have renewed your commitment to eat healthier. Each breath you take increases the good confident feelings within.
3. You feel more in balance, in perfect harmony with your renewed body & emotions and at peace of mind, body, heart and soul. Now you are experiencing an everlasting state of gratitude for your empowered life.
4. Feeling vibrant, energized and refreshed as you move to full alertness.
5. You can open your eyes with a new sense of joy, profound happiness and contentment."

GLOSSARY:

Autosuggestion - Giving oneself positive suggestion such as with self-hypnosis, self- healing and affirmations.

Cellular Memory - A physical response resulting from an emotional memory, such as in a psychosomatic illness.

Hypnosis - An experience resulting from profound relaxation when a person's concentration has narrowed down to what is being heard, seen, felt or experienced in a way that is unique to each person.

Hypnotherapy - The use of hypnosis for the purpose of therapy.

Hypnotic Induction - suggestions designed to promote profound relaxation in short or long form.

Hypnotic Prescription - a series of suggestions that are designed to assist in helping client achieve their goal.

Hypnotherapy Session - A session usually between 25 and 40 minutes wherein a person or a group is guided by a hypnotherapist. This session includes induction, deepening, acceptance, resolution of cause and awakening.

Post Hypnotic Suggestion - is specifically designed to be effective after hypnotic session is finished.

Conscious Level of Mind - awareness of those thoughts we can easily recall. The part of the mind we consciously use in our daily life for thinking.

Subconscious Level of Mind - information that can be recalled using an altered state such as in hypnosis, self-hypnosis, guided imagery. Everything that has occurred from birth to present that we normally don't recollect on a conscious level.

Books by Art Winkler & Pam Winkler

Get Rid of Fat Forever

Hypnosis

Overcome Psychosomatic Illness Through Hypnosis

The Power of Suggestion with Hypnosis

Mind Medicine

St. John's University

www.sjunow.org

Self-Help

ABOUT THE AUTHOR

Carol Cumpston studied hypnotherapy at St. John's University receiving her BS cum laude in 1995. She has been a lifelong learner and hypnotherapist and developed a weight reduction series, smoking cessation, stress management and quick recovery from surgery plus more.